Copyright © 2021 by I LEWIS

All rights reserved. No part of this publication may be reproduced, distributed, or transmitted in any form or by any means, including photocopying, recording, or other electronic or mechanical methods, without the prior written permission of the publisher, except in the case of brief quotation embodied in critical reviews and certain other non-commercial uses permitted by copyright law.

Table of Contents

Introduction 3

History Of Kombucha 8

What Is Kombucha? 31

Composition and properties of Kombucha 32

Health Claims 39

Kombucha Health Benefits 44

Available Flavors of Kombucha 61

Frequently Asked Questions 65

How To Make Kombucha Tea at Home 74

Conclusion 86

Introduction

Kombucha tea is a slightly sweet, slightly acidic refreshing beverage consumed worldwide. It is obtained from infusion of tea leaves by the fermentation of a symbiotic association of bacteria and yeasts forming "tea fungus" (Chen and Liu 2000). A floating cellulosic pellicle layer and the sour liquid broth are the 2 portions of kombucha tea. It tastes like sparkling apple cider and can be produced in the home by fermentation using mail order or locally available tea fungus. Though green tea can be used for kombucha preparation, black tea and white sugar are considered the finest substrates. Kombucha is the internationally used Germanized form of the Japanese name for this slightly fermented tea beverage. It was first used in East Asia for its healing benefits. Kombucha originated in northeast China (Manchuria) where it was prized during the Tsin Dynasty ("Ling Chi"), about 220 B.C., for its detoxifying and energizing properties. In 414 A.D., the physician Kombu brought the tea fungus to Japan and he used it to cure the digestive problems of the Emperor Inkyo. As trade routes expanded, kombucha (former trade name "Mo-Gu") found its way first into Russian (as Cainiigrib, Cainii kvass, Japonskigrib, Kambucha, Jsakvasska) and then into other eastern European areas, appearing in Germany (as Heldenpilz, Kombuchaschwamm) around the turn of the 20th century. During World War II, this beverage was again introduced into Germany, and in the 1950's it arrived in France and also in France-dominated North Africa where its consumption became quite popular. The habit of drinking fermented tea became acceptable throughout

Europe until World War II which brought widespread shortages of the necessary tea leaves and sugar. In the postwar years, Italian society's passion for the beverage (called "Funkochinese") peaked in the 1950s. In the 1960s, science researchers in Switzerland reported that drinking kombucha was similarly beneficial as eating yogurt and kombucha's popularity increased. Today, kombucha is sold worldwide in retail food stores in different flavors and kombucha culture is sold in several online shopping websites. A kombucha journal is electronically published by Gunther W. Frank and available worldwide in 30 languages (Dufresne and Farnworth 2000; Hartmann and others 2000).

Kombucha is a semi-sweet, semi-sour, sometimes effervescent drink that you can make at home for pennies, and with minimal equipment and skill.

I recently drove cross-country for a summer vacation and was asked to teach an intro class to kombucha for beginners at my hometown library. I've been brewing kombucha on and off for a few years, and am certainly no expert, but of course I said sure! And then started thinking about the logistics of transporting the needed bits and bobs. It was a bit of a gong show, but ultimately worked out nicely, and now there are twelve new brewers enjoying this delicious drink.

In getting ready to teach the kombucha for beginners class though, I found myself doing some reading and research and have put it all together here. I was surprised to learn of the mysterious and undocumented history of this drink.

History Of Kombucha

Once dubbed the most liberal product in America in 2009, kombucha is experiencing a surge of sales and quickly becoming an influential player in the domestic beverage economy. The misunderstood ancient fermented beverage has a complicated history in terms of media perception, alcoholic regulation and availability of human-based medical studies. However, big business is taking note of the developing consumer preferences for the functional beverage and its noted health benefits. So how did this ancient Chinese beverage that is brewed with an unappetizing yeast disc become an artisanal beverage and an influential part of PepsiCo's brand portfolio in 2016? How was it possible that an alcohol regulation scandal in 2010 inversely generated huge consumer interest for the product? To understand its current state and growing market potential, a critical lens should be given to the drink's long history and its surprising informative pivots.

Kombucha tea, the brew is ready to be placed in storage with the bacteria culture in place to ferment the brew.

HOW IT'S MADE

If you are not familiar, kombucha is a fermented and sweetened tea often made with black or green tea. It is largely classified as a functional beverage, meaning that it is a non-alcoholic drink that contains vitamins, amino acids or other nutrients associated with health benefits. The process of preparing kombucha can vary but generally involves a double fermentation process wherein a

SCOBY (a pancake-shaped symbiotic culture of bacteria and yeast) is placed in a sweetened tea mixture and left to ferment at room temperature for 1-3 weeks, and then bottled for 1-2 weeks to contain released CO_2 and encourage carbonation. From there, bottled kombucha is placed in a refrigerated environment to slow down the carbonation and fermentation processes. Lack of awareness around this second fermentation cycle led to misregulation of alcohol content in recent years. Additionally, the antimicrobial properties of this process make its production process sanitary and safe for homebrewing.

HISTORY (200 B.C. - 2010)

Kombucha originated in Northeast China (historically referred to as Manchuria) around 220

B.C. and was initially prized for its healing properties. Its name is reportedly derived from Dr. Kombu, a Korean physician who brought the fermented tea to Japan as a curative for Emperor Inkyo. Eventually the tea was brought to Europe as a result of trade route expansions in the early 20th century, most notably appearing in Russia (as "Kambucha") and Germany (as "Kombuchaschwamm"). Despite a dip in international popularity during WWII due to the shortage of tea and sugar supplies, kombucha regained popularity following a 1960s study in Switzerland comparing its health benefits to those of yogurt.

Kombucha most meaningfully gained popularity in domestic markets in the 1990s. Sandor Katz, a leading fermentation expert and author of The Art of Fermentation, noted that this initial popularity was due in part to consumers who believed that the beverage was a powerful health aid for serious medical conditions. Katz explained, "I first tried kombucha around 1994, when a friend of mine with AIDS started making and drinking it as a health practice. It was touted as a general immune stimulant, though claims of kombucha's benefits have been extraordinarily varied and broad."

Initially kombucha in the United States was distributed solely by grassroots efforts wherein enthusiasts would share their SCOBYs (a symbiotic culture of bacteria and yeast disc) with others so that they could homebrew the tea themselves. Many attribute the formal start of the domestic kombucha industry to GT Dave who founded GT's Kombucha, which has continued to be the leading domestic kombucha brand. GT's Kombucha began in 1995 as a mission-driven family business that initially sold to local health stores before gaining widespread popularity.

Much like the anecdote of Sandor Katz's friend, Dave partially credits his passion for kombucha to his belief that it cured his mother's cancer. The GT's Kombucha website still explicitly cites this claim: "In 1995, my life came crashing down when I heard that my mother, Laraine had just been diagnosed with a highly aggressive form of breast cancer. After a week of emotional turmoil, I was relieved to find out that her breast cancer had not spread and that the pungent tasting cultured tea that she had been drinking was part of the reason why." Memorial Sloan Kettering Cancer Center notes that kombucha tea has not been shown to treat cancer or AIDS in humans.

Studies conducted through 2010 suggested that the health benefit anecdotes associated with kombucha have occasionally been overblown by the media and industry figureheads, due to overbiasing positive results from nonhuman studies and anecdotal human studies. However, researchers believe that kombucha's tea base and fermentation process imply that the beverage contains similar benefits to plain tea and fermented foods, including probiotic benefits that encourage gut bacteria diversity and aid digestion.

An employee of BAO Food and Drink, a manufacturer of organic fermented foods, fills bottles of... kombucha in their bottling space at the Organic Food Incubator in Long Island City, in the Queens borough of New York, U.S., on Wednesday,

July 16, 2014. The 20,000 square foot space offers commercial kitchens for small companies producing natural products.

2010 REGULATION CRISIS

Through the early 2000s, kombucha continued to see healthy growth due in part to increased consumer awareness via expanded grassroots distribution and the increased availability of GT's Kombucha. However, the production and distribution of kombucha halted abruptly for two months in 2010 following a Whole Foods inspection by Maine Department of Agriculture Consumer Protection Inspector Randy Trahan. During a routine bottle audit at the Whole Foods in Portland, Trahan noticed leaking kombucha bottles. Trahan explained, "Some of the Kombucha bottles on the shelf were leaking. Being a public health official, I know that alcohol is a by-product of the fermentation process. I could immediately see that there might be a public safety issue...Kids could get hold of this and get a buzz."

Trahan submitted a few of the store's bottles for testing at the Food Sciences Lab at The University of Maine where it was discovered that the bottles contained alcohol levels ranging from slightly over 0.5% to over 2.5%, which was well above the Alcohol and Tobacco Tax and Trade Bureau's regulation that labeled non-alcoholic beverages must contain less than 0.5% ABV. This suggests that many producers were not taking precaution to halt or account for the continued ABV development during kombucha's second fermentation and bottling, and that regulators had a lack of awareness about kombucha's second fermentation.

Shortly after the analysis results had been released, Whole Foods removed kombucha from its shelves on June 15, 2010 alongside a display note that read, "Key suppliers and Whole Foods Market have elected to voluntarily withdraw kombucha products in bottles and on tap from our stores at this time due to labeling concerns related to slightly elevated alcohol levels in some products. This is not a quality issue. Sorry for any inconvenience."

NEW STANDARDS AND REGULATIONS

In response to the falsely labeled alcohol content on some kombucha bottles, the Alcohol and

Tobacco Tax and Trade Bureau updated its guidelines to highlight that that it would regulate any kombucha products that contain 0.5% or more ABV, even after the product was bottled and continued to ferment.

Around this time, kombucha expert Hannah Crum also helped to co-found Kombucha Brewers International, a trade association for commercial kombucha brewers that aimed to educate consumers and retailers about kombucha as well as promote industry ethics and labeling standards. KBI was the first kombucha organization that could act as a third party to work directly with regulators without the biased perspective that may have been associated with advocacy from conversations held by a single brand. Crum noted, "It was clear as a result that most government agencies and businesses don't want to hear the point of view from the brand. So if you can create an industry hub where the information comes from the broader industry and not just the brand, it has a lot more weight." KBI has since worked closely with regulators to help create a standardized alcohol content test and a quality verification process.

Once new regulations were in development, kombucha producers diverged into two paths as a result: some complied with the ABV guidelines through various changes to their manufacturing processes, while others stuck to their original formulas which measured above 0.5% ABV and some even created consciously-labeled kombucha beer brands. Those who decided to decrease their ABV used a combination of de-alcoholizers, alterations to recipes and sugar content, yeast manipulation and more.

POST-2010 RECOVERY AND GROWTH

During the two month production break, the kombucha industry was also hit with an associated outbreak of media confusion about kombucha's alcohol content due to allegations that Lindsay Lohan's alcohol-monitoring bracelet was set off in July of 2010 due to the star's regular consumption of kombucha.

Despite the distribution halt and seemingly negative media coverage, there was an increase in consumer awareness and demand for the product which led to a 28% category sales increase YoY through June 2011. Leading kombucha industry expert and co-founder of the Kombucha Brewers Guild, Hannah Crum, spoke with a number of kombucha companies shortly thereafter and noted, "Nearly all Kombucha companies interviewed agreed that the difficulties of last summer generated more consumer interest and led to expansion rather than contraction." She added that existing kombucha fans could have helped this increase in sales due to their strong product loyalty and increasing fandom bred by diminished availability. She added, "Most fans spent the summer wondering not why it was removed, but obsessing over how and when it would be coming back."

Additionally, the removal of major brands like GT's Kombucha from the shelves of national retailers resulted in the visibility and growth of smaller, regional kombucha brands, like Buchi. In an interview with Hannah Crum, Jeannine Bucher of Buchi stated, "Because we self-distribute, the national distribution withdrawal was a golden opportunity for us to introduce Buchi to Kombucha drinkers whose national brand was no longer available."

As many brands altered their recipes, there were mixed reactions from longtime kombucha fans who believed that these new de-alcoholizaition processes minimized the health benefits of kombucha as well as negatively impacted the taste. As a result, some producers continued to produce their original unadulterated kombucha formulas which contained above 0.5% ABV and have them regulated by the Alcohol and Tobacco Tax and Trade Bureau and shelved accordingly in stores. However, this awareness of the health benefits of undoctored kombucha and its potential alcohol content led way to the creation of a new kombucha beverage segment: kombucha beer.

A number of kombucha beer brands have since arose in recent years. Unlike kombucha that adheres to the 0.5% non-alcoholic guidelines, kombucha beer is typically allowed to naturally ferment for longer periods of time through its second fermentation and then not pasteurized, preserving much of its live bacteria and associated health properties. Kombucha beer is consciously marketed as a healthier alternative to traditional beers based on its lower caloric contents and gluten-free properties, as well as being positioned as an artisanal beverage.

One of the leaders in this new segment is Kombrewcha, a New York City based brand founded in November of 2014. Founded by Barry Nalebuff, co-founder of Honest Tea and a professor at the Yale School of Management, and Ariel Glazer, a natural foods entrepreneur and former Goldman Sachs analyst, the pair sought to create a tea-based beverage that was low in both calories and alcohol content. Kombrewcha contains 65-75 calories, 4-6 grams of sugar and 2% ABV and is naturally gluten-free because it is made from tea as well as contains live probiotics.

Kristina Marino, Kombrewcha's Director of Marketing, explained how their product is fundamentally different from those in the non-alcoholic kombucha and alcoholic beverage markets: "The problem we saw is that alcoholic beverages—mixed drinks, beer, and hard cider—are either too high in alcohol and calories or too low in taste. A regular 12 oz beer ranges from about 140 calories to over 300 calories, same for hard cider - mixed drinks often have more than 300 calories. Even light beers typically have over 100 calories."

Additionally, Kombrewcha is departing from the traditional alternative health image of kombucha by conciously positioning itself as an artisanal beverage. The brand has partnered with a number of highly regarded restaurants and bars across New York to serve and increase exposure for the brand, including Murray's Cheese Bar, Roebling Tea Room and Angelica Kitchen. A number of these establishments also serve Kombrewcha-based cocktails, such as Meadowsweet's Kombrewcha Mule.

Kombrewcha has experienced profound growth and expansion since its 2014 debut, indicating that consumers are responsive to the concept of kombucha beer. In 2016, the brand's sales increased 40% YoY and the brand plans to launch on the West Coast in 2017.

Across all segments of kombucha, the beverage saw impressive growth and sales through 2016. Errol Schweizer, executive global grocery coordinator for Whole Foods Market, noted that kombucha occupies up to one-third of refrigerated functional-beverage shelf space in Whole Foods stores. Additionally, US consumers purchased almost $400 million in kombucha in 2014, compared to its 2010 sales of a little more than $100 million during the aformentioned 2010 regulation crisis.

KOMBUCHA'S FUTURE

Despite its 2010 regulation crisis and rippling product confusion among consumers, kombucha sales are stronger than ever and projected to keep growing. Kombucha is considered the fastest-growing product in the functional beverage market with sales estimates of $1.8 billion by 2020. Additionally, domestic kombucha sales have a CAGR of 25.0% between 2015 to 2020. Analysts believe this is due in part to the new alcoholic segment of the kombucha market, like the aforementioned unadultered kombuchas and kombucha beers.

Most recently, PepsiCo has taken notice of the promising future of kombucha with its purchase of leading kombucha brand KeVita in November 2016. An announcement posted on the PepsiCo website on November 22, 2016 by Chris Lansing, PepsiCo Premium Nutrition's general manager and vice president, explained, "I am pleased to welcome KeVita into the PepsiCo family. Under the leadership of CEO Bill Moses, KeVita has become an innovative, high-growth brand that is transforming the functional beverage space... This announcement is further evidence of PepsiCo's focus on delivering Performance with Purpose by continuing to evolve our health and wellness offerings to meet consumers' changing needs."

KeVita will join PepsiCo's 22 global brands that are purchased by consumers one billion times a day in over 200 countries. This move is a strong signal of market confidence in kombucha's growth potential, in particular because Pepsi has a history of investing in multiple long term horizons, regardless of conflicting present consumer sentiment. Pepsi CEO Indra Nooyi recently explained the company's investment strategy alongside another controversial announcement that the company may eventually invest in bug proteins. Nooyi stated, "One year, three year, five year, ten year: we have different people looking at different horizons, because if you believe in the ten year horizons and what we are seeing, some of the weirdest food and beverage habits are showing up."

Kombucha's strong future is evident, and perhaps best compared to the popularity arc of yogurt. Hannah Crum explains this belief within the kombucha industry when she stated, "We consider ourselves the 21st century yogurt. In our parents' generation, you had to make your own yogurt because it wasn't a commercial product, but then people heard the health benefits and how it could extend your life and then it became a multi-million dollar industry. We think people in the future will grow up just accepting kombucha as a product they had as a kid."

What Is Kombucha?

Kombucha is a fizzy sweet-and-sour drink made with tea. Many people say it helps relieve or prevent a variety of health problems, everything from hair loss to cancer and AIDS. There's little scientific evidence to back up the claims, but some elements of the drink may be good for you.

Composition and properties of Kombucha

Biological

A kombucha culture is a symbiotic culture of bacteria and yeast (SCOBY), similar to mother of vinegar, containing one or more species each of bacteria and yeasts, which form a zoogleal mat known as a "mother". There is a broad spectrum of yeast species spanning several genera reported to be present in kombucha culture including species of Zygosaccharomyces, Candida, Kloeckera/Hanseniaspora, Torulaspora, Pichia, Brettanomyces/Dekkera, Saccharomyces, Lachancea, Saccharomycoides, Schizosaccharomyces, and Kluyveromyces.

The bacterial component of kombucha comprises several species, almost always including Komagataeibacter xylinus (formerly Gluconacetobacter xylinus), which ferments alcohols produced by the yeasts into acetic and other acids, increasing the acidity and limiting ethanol content. The bacteria of kombucha require large amounts of oxygen for their growth and activity. The population of bacteria and yeasts found to produce acetic acid has been reported to increase for the first 4 days of fermentation, decreasing thereafter. K. xylinus has been shown to produce microbial cellulose, and is reportedly responsible for most or all of the physical structure of the "mother", which may have been selectively encouraged over time for firmer (denser) and more robust cultures by brewers.

The mixed, presumably symbiotic culture has been further described as being lichenous, in accord with the reported presence of the known lichenous natural product usnic acid, though as of 2015, no report appears indicating the standard cyanobacterial species of lichens in association with kombucha fungal components.

Chemical composition

Kombucha is made by adding the kombucha culture into a broth of sugared tea. The sugar serves as a nutrient for the SCOBY that allows for bacterial growth in the tea. Sucrose is converted, biochemically, into fructose and glucose, and these into gluconic acid and acetic acid. In addition, kombucha contains enzymes and amino acids, polyphenols, and various other organic acids which vary between preparations. Other specific components include ethanol (see below), glucuronic acid, glycerol, lactic acid, usnic acid (a hepatotoxin, see above), and B-vitamins. Kombucha has also been found to contain vitamin C.

The alcohol content of kombucha is usually less than 0.5%, but increases with extended fermentation times. Over-fermentation generates high amounts of acids similar to vinegar. The pH of the drink is typically about 3.5.

Production Of Kombucha

Kombucha can be prepared at home or commercially. Kombucha is made by dissolving sugar in non-chlorinated boiling water. Tea leaves are steeped in the hot sugar water and discarded. The sweetened tea is cooled and the SCOBY culture is added. The mixture is then poured into a sterilized beaker along with previously fermented kombucha tea to lower the pH. The container is covered with a paper towel or breathable fabric to prevent insects such as fruit flies from contaminating the kombucha.

The tea is left to ferment for a period of up to 10 to 14 days at room temperature (18 °C to 26 °C). A new "daughter" SCOBY will form on the surface of the tea to the diameter of the container. After fermentation is completed, the SCOBY is removed and stored along with a small amount of the newly fermented tea. The remaining kombucha is strained and bottled for a secondary ferment for a few days or stored at a temperature of 4°C.

Commercially bottled kombucha became available in the late 1990s. In 2010, elevated alcohol levels were found in many bottled kombucha products, leading retailers including Whole Foods to temporarily pull the drinks from store shelves. In response, kombucha suppliers reformulated their products to have lower alcohol levels.

By 2014, US sales of bottled kombucha were $400 million, $350 million of which was earned by Millennium Products, Inc. which sells GT's Kombucha. In 2014, the companies that make and sell kombucha formed a trade organization, Kombucha Brewers International. In 2016, PepsiCo purchased kombucha maker KeVita for approximately $200 million. In the US, sales of kombucha and other fermented drinks rose by 37 percent in 2017. Beer companies like Full Sail Brewing Company and Molson Coors Beverage Company produce kombucha by themselves or via subsidiaries.

Hard kombucha

As of 2019, some commercial kombucha producers sell "hard kombucha" with an alcohol content of over 5 percent. Brands include Boochcraft, June Shine, and Kombrewcha.

Health Claims

Many people drink kombucha tea for its purported health benefits. There have not been any human trials conducted to assess its possible biological effects, and the purported health benefits resulting from its biological activities have not been demonstrated in humans. A 2003 systematic review characterized kombucha as an "extreme example" of an unconventional remedy because of the disparity between implausible, wide-ranging health claims and the potential risks of the product. It concluded that the proposed, unsubstantiated therapeutic claims did not outweigh known risks, and that kombucha should not be recommended for therapeutic use, being in a class of "remedies that only seem to benefit those who sell them."

Adverse effects

Reports of adverse effects related to kombucha consumption are rare, but may be underreported, according to the 2003 review. The American Cancer Society says that "Serious side effects and occasional deaths have been associated with drinking Kombucha tea". Because kombucha is a commonly homemade fermentation, caution should be taken because pathogenic microorganisms can contaminate the tea during preparation.

Adverse effects associated with kombucha consumption include severe hepatic (liver) and renal (kidney) toxicity as well as metabolic acidosis. At least one person is known to have died after consuming kombucha, though the drink itself has never been conclusively proven as the cause of death.

Some adverse health effects may arise from the acidity of the tea causing acidosis, and brewers are cautioned to avoid over-fermentation. Other adverse effects may be a result of bacterial or fungal contamination during the brewing process. Some studies have found the hepatotoxin usnic acid in kombucha, although it is not known whether the cases of liver damage are due to usnic acid or to some other toxin.

Drinking kombucha can be harmful for people with preexisting ailments. Due to its microbial sourcing and possible non-sterile packaging, kombucha is not recommended for people with poor immune function women who are pregnant or nursing, or children under 4 years old. It may compromise immune responses or stomach acidity in these susceptible populations. There are certain drugs that one should not take at the same time as kombucha because of the small percentage of alcohol content.

A 2019 systematic review confirmed the numerous health risks, but said "kombucha is not considered harmful if about 4 US fluid ounces (120 ml) per day is consumed by healthy individuals; potential risks are associated with a low pH brew leaching heavy metals from containers, excessive consumption of highly acidic kombucha, or consumption by individuals with pre-existing health conditions."

Kombucha Ingredients

The basic ingredients in kombucha are yeast, sugar, and black tea. The mix is set aside for a week or more. During that time, bacteria and acids form in the drink, as well as a small amount of alcohol. This process is known as fermentation, and it's similar to how cabbage is preserved as sauerkraut or kimchi, or how milk is turned into yogurt.

These bacteria and acids form a film on top of the liquid called a SCOBY (symbiotic colony of bacteria and yeast). You can use a SCOBY to ferment more kombucha.

Kombucha bacteria includes lactic-acid bacteria, which can work as a probiotic. Kombucha also contains a healthy dose of B vitamins.

Kombucha Health Benefits

Advocates say it helps your digestion, rids your body of toxins, and boosts your energy. It's also said to boost your immune system, help you lose weight, ward off high blood pressure and heart disease, and prevent cancer. But there's not a lot of evidence to support these claims.

Claims about kombucha's power to aid digestion come from the fact that fermentation makes probiotics. Probiotics help with diarrhea and irritable bowel syndrome (IBS), and they may even strengthen your immune system.

When kombucha is made from green tea, you get its benefits, too. This includes bioactive compounds, such as polyphenols, that act as antioxidants. Antioxidants protect your cells from damage.

Green tea may also help you burn fat and protect you from heart disease. Studies in animals show that the drink lowers cholesterol and blood sugar levels, among other things. But research hasn't shown that it has the same effects in people.

Nonetheless, early research suggests it may boost your gut health and more. Here's a glance at the potential benefits that researchers continue to explore.

1. **May Help Boost Metabolism**

    If you're looking to drop a few extra pounds, you'll likely consider anything that'll jump-start your metabolism.

Kombucha isn't a miracle weight loss drink. But thanks to the epigallocatechin-3-gallate (EGCG) found in the green tea of some types of kombucha, it may be a secret to a slightly faster metabolism.

EGCG is a catechin, a compound found in green tea. According to a review published in May 2017 in the Journal of Nutritional Biochemistry, catechins have the potential to boost metabolic rates in adults. But existing studies on the topic are short and small, and the authors of the review note that more research is needed to know the true effects of EGCG on metabolism.

2. **May Aid Constipation**

As a potential source of probiotics, one purported health benefit of kombucha is its ability to balance good bacteria in the gut and relieve some gastrointestinal issues, but more research is needed, according to the Cleveland Clinic.

An study published in April 2014 in Food Microbiology examined the microbial components of kombucha and identified a "prominent lactobacillus population" in the drink. Lactobacillus is a common type of probiotic, so it's plausible that kombucha may stabilize the digestive tract and help prevent infections and inflammation. And if so, drinking kombucha might improve irritable bowel syndrome, inflammatory bowel diseases, bloating, and constipation, notes the Cleveland Clinic.

3. **May Reduce Inflammation**

Chronic inflammation is involved in just about every health condition, including heart disease, diabetes, arthritis, allergies, and respiratory illnesses such as chronic obstructive pulmonary disease (COPD), according to a June 2019 article in StatPearls

Kombucha isn't a first-line choice for treating any chronic disease, but the drink may complement your healthy diet, lifestyle choices, and medication regimen. That's because the teas used to make kombucha contain polyphenols, which are antioxidants that can lessen inflammation in the body, according to the Journal of Chemistry review.

There's also a growing belief in the scientific community that eating gut-friendly foods may help lower inflammation in the intestinal tract, and for this in particular, kombucha may be helpful, notes a review published in February 2015 in Microbial Ecology in Health and Disease.

Inflammation is at the root of some gastrointestinal conditions, such as inflammatory bowel diseases, and research suggests that low-grade inflammation might contribute to irritable bowel syndrome. This inflammation may be the result of an imbalance of good and bad bacteria in the gut, known as gut dysbiosis. The idea is that when bad bacteria overtake the good, this triggers an immune system response, and it's this response that leads to inflammation, suggests the Microbial Ecology in Health and Disease review.

4. **May Play a Role in Helping Prevent Cancer**

There's also growing evidence that kombucha may assist with the prevention of certain types of cancer, although more research is needed. This claim is based on kombucha having antioxidant properties, which help rid the body of free radicals and other harmful substances that promote the growth of cancerous cells, notes the review in the Journal of Nutritional Biochemistry.

A study published in the January-February 2013 issue of Biomedicine & Preventive Nutrition found that kombucha inhibits angiogenesis, which the National Cancer Institute explains is the growth of new blood vessels. The study highlighted that prostate cancer is angiogenesis-dependent, meaning that new blood cells can feed and contribute to the growth of these tumors. By inhibiting angiogenesis, researchers concluded that kombucha could help decrease the survival of prostate cancer cells. Of course, more research is needed.

Per the Journal of Nutritional Biochemistry review, the compounds in kombucha that may help inhibit cancer growth include polyphenols, gluconic acid, glucuronic acid, lactic acid, and vitamin C.

5. **May Help Strengthen the Immune System**

The gut-healthy benefits of kombucha may also provide an immune system boost. It's important to note that the digestive system and immune system are closely intertwined; the lining of the intestines creates antibodies that help protect the body, according to John Hopkins Medicine. A huge portion of the immune system is found in the gut, more specifically about 70 percent, according to a study.

Thus, Zenhausern explains, optimal gut health is the key to a strong immune system. The fermenting bacteria in kombucha can boost immunity, thanks to the dose of good bacteria they provide, says Zenhausern.

6. **May Aid Depression Treatment**

Symptoms of depression vary from person to person but can include a general feeling of sadness and hopelessness.

Depression can also cause problems, including insomnia, poor concentration, and low energy, according to the Mayo Clinic. But kombucha might provide some relief, helping boost your mood by cranking up the production of feel-good hormones, such as serotonin, notes the Mayo Clinic.

There haven't been studies specifically linking kombucha and depression. But a February 2017 review published in the Annals of General Psychiatry does suggest that some psychiatric disorders may be connected with changes in the microbiome (the environment of bacteria in the gut), so there's increasing evidence that probiotics may help relieve symptoms of depression and anxiety.

Zenhausern further notes that 95 percent of serotonin is produced in your gut, not your brain, so optimal gut health is important for mental health and mood regulation, too.

"This is why it is always important to address gut health when boosting mood and fighting against depression," she says.

7. **May Boost Cardiovascular Health**

According to the Centers for Disease Control and Prevention (CDC), heart disease increases the risk of stroke or heart attack, but healthy lifestyle changes can improve your cardiovascular health.

This includes following a healthy diet high in vegetables, fruits, whole grains, and lean proteins. You should also incorporate exercise, medication, and yes, even kombucha.

The potential benefit is in kombucha's possible ability to positively influence cholesterol levels, according to the Journal of Chemistry research. High cholesterol is one factor for heart disease, notes the CDC.

Researchers need to conduct more human studies to confirm the effectiveness of kombucha on cholesterol.

But according to a study published in April 2015 in Pharmaceutical Biology, rats administered kombucha showed lower levels of LDL ("bad") cholesterol) and higher levels of HDL ("good") cholesterol). More research is needed, but future studies could similarly reveal that kombucha improves cholesterol levels in humans. Only time will tell.

8. **May Promote Liver Health**

Similarly, kombucha may improve liver health due to its potential ability to detoxify the body. So over time, drinking the beverage may reduce how hard your liver has to work, per the Journal of Chemistry.

In the Pharmaceutical Biology study, rats administered kombucha also showed decreased levels of thiobarbituric acid reactive substances in their livers. This organic compound is a measure of cell and tissue damage. Still, more clinical research is needed to know whether the benefit holds up.

9. May Play a Role in Lowering Blood Sugar

Drinking kombucha might also benefit those who are insulin resistant or have diabetes. The tea can inhibit α-amylase, a protein in the pancreas that's responsible for higher postprandial (after meal) glucose levels, per a study.

According to the Pharmaceutical Biology study, kombucha had a curative effect on rats with diabetes after 30 days, and it also improved their liver and kidney function

More research is needed, but the findings suggest that kombucha could one day be used as a complementary treatment for diabetes, in addition to traditional approaches, including weight loss, diet, exercise, oral medications, and insulin.

10. Help Maintain Healthy Weight

Kombucha can be an alternative drink if you enjoy soda or juices yet are looking for a beverage with fewer calories and less sugar and to lose or maintain your weight.

Sugar is high in empty calories, and when consumed in excess, there's the risk of taking in more calories than you burn, resulting in weight gain.

Remember, kombucha isn't sugar-free (most of the sugar is fermented, but some remains in the final product). Even so, a typical drink may have only 6 to 8 grams (g) per serving, says Rebecca Stib, RDN, who's based in Boston and is the cofounder of Nutritious Gifts. "You'll have to double the amount for brands that have two servings in a bottle, but it's still lower than your typical serving of a can of soda or juice drink, which can be upward of 25 g per serving," warns Stib.

For comparison's sake, a bottle of organic, raw kombucha can have 30 calories and 8 g of sugar in 8 ounces, per the website for GTS, a kombucha brand. On the other hand, 8 ounces of soda can have 60 calories and 16 g of sugar, according to the Coca-Cola website

Available Flavors of Kombucha

Fortunately, if you want to give kombucha a try, you don't have to make your own — but this is an option, too.

Kombucha is available at health-food stores, grocery stores, and online. You'll find a variety of flavors to tempt your taste buds. Examples include these kombucha flavors:

- Ginger
- Green tea
- Raspberry
- Blueberry
- Dragonfruit
- Lemon

Is There Sugar in Kombucha?

Although some brands of kombucha have very little sugar in their products, some manufacturers add flavor, juice, and higher amounts of sugar during the preparation stage, for taste and sweetness. There aren't specific guidelines on how much sugar is too much in a bottle of kombucha, so you'll have to use your discretion.

Yet Casey Seiden, RD, who is based in New York City, encourages consumers to look at drinks like kombucha in the context of their added sugar intake throughout the day. "If you've already guzzled another sugary drink and had extra sweets, then perhaps limit yourself to one kombucha," she warns. The American Heart Association recommends consuming no more than 6 teaspoons (equal to 25 grams or 100 calories) of added sugar per day for women. Men are allowed a bit more — about 9 teaspoons (equal to 36 g or 150 calories) of added sugar per day, per the organization.

Kombucha Risks

Making kombucha involves letting bacteria grow in a liquid you're going to drink. Many of the bacteria are considered probiotics, but if it's not prepared properly, it can grow harmful bacteria or mold.

Since the mid-1990s, several cases of illness and at least one death have been reported in people who drank kombucha. Ailments included liver problems, lactic acidosis (a buildup of lactic acid in the body), allergic reactions, and nausea.

The nonprofit product research group Consumer Reports advises against drinking it because of the risk of contamination and little proof of benefits.

But the FDA says kombucha is safe when properly prepared. If you're making it at home, experts recommend using glass, stainless steel, or plastic containers. Keep everything sanitary, including the equipment and your hands.

Frequently Asked Questions

Is kombucha good for digestion?

Foods that go through a natural fermentation process gain probiotic properties, and eating these foods may bring benefits like improved digestion and a more balanced gut microbiome. Many nutritionists believe kombucha may be beneficial to gut health due to these probiotics, though they say more research is needed.

"Some sources claim that kombucha can positively impact gut health [by] decreasing inflammation and providing antioxidants because of the probiotics, however more research needs to be completed to confirm this claim," says Tracy

Lockwood Beckerman, a registered dietitian in New York City.

Maria Zamarripa, a Denver-based registered dietitian, says kombucha and its beneficial probiotics can support gut health, but she stresses that the drink is not a substitute for a healthy diet. "Consuming a diet rich in fiber from fruits, vegetables, nuts and seeds is the most important factor in order to promote a healthy gut environment for these probiotics to flourish," she says.

Does kombucha have caffeine?

Kombucha usually contains a bit of caffeine (since it's made with tea), but the amount is small when compared to coffee, tea, soda and other popular caffeinated beverages. Typically, about one-third of the tea's caffeine remains after it's been fermented, which is about 10 to 25 milligrams per serving for black tea, says Colleen Chiariello, chief clinical dietitian in the department of food and nutrition at Syosset Hospital in New York. This is generally not enough caffeine to have an impact on most people, but the response can vary from person to person.

How much alcohol is in kombucha?

All kombucha contains a small amount of alcohol that is created during the fermentation process, but usually it's not enough for a person to feel its effects. The commercially available varieties sold in the U.S. must contain less than 0.5% alcohol by volume to be sold as non-alcoholic beverages, as mandated by the Alcohol and Tobacco Tax and

Trade Bureau. (A beer typically contains around 5% alcohol, and a 5-ounce glass of wine has around 12% alcohol.)

Is kombucha bad for your teeth?

Kombucha's acidity is potentially problematic, but further studies are needed to learn more about how the drink impacts oral health. "We can speculate that kombucha's low pH, which is similar to that of soda, can have a comparable effect," says Clarisa Amarillas Gastelum, assistant professor in the Department of General Dentistry at Stony Brook School of Dental Medicine.

Low pH beverages may compromise the tooth enamel and increase the likelihood of tooth discoloration when drinking highly pigmented beverages, she says. But this doesn't necessarily mean you need to ditch kombucha altogether. To protect your teeth, Gastelum recommends drinking your kombucha in one sitting rather than sipping throughout the day, using a straw and rinsing your mouth with water after finishing.

Is it safe to drink kombucha regularly?

Nutrition experts say it's fine for most people to sip on kombucha every day, but to check with your doctor if you're unsure about drinking it. Some recommend that pregnant or breastfeeding women and people with compromised immune systems should stay away from kombucha because the drink's live bacteria could be harmful.

"When you are pregnant or you are in an immunocompromised condition, those live bacteria can get into your blood, causing disease," Li says. "It's almost the same as when we tell a pregnant woman and immunocompromised patient don't eat raw fish. That's the same concern."

Be mindful of how much you drink, too. "Some people may not tolerate large amounts of kombucha right away," Zamarripa says. "Start by drinking 4 ounces or less per day, and increase the volume based on your tolerance."

Can kombucha harm you?

"Commercial products should be safe," Dr. Walton Sumner, a research scholar with the Ronin Institute and a co-author of the review on the available literature.said. "But you probably don't want to use it for all your hydration." He also advises to drink it in moderation.

There are some exclusions: those with kidney or lung disease, who are at risk for acidosis, a condition in which there is too much acid in the blood. In 1995, two Iowa women fell critically ill after drinking homemade kombucha, and one of them died. Also, the Scoby can cause an infection in those who are immunosuppressed.

The sugar content can also be high for those watching their intake. Be aware of the range: from five grams a serving (Better Booch's Rose Bliss) to 14 grams (Wonder Drink's Asian Pear & Ginger).

The shifting levels of alcohol in kombucha can pose a problem for pregnant women, children, and individuals with liver disease or pancreatitis or those in recovery.

"Given that alcohol is a substance with well documented harms, the label should feature a clear and prominent indication of alcohol content," Dr. Anna Lembke, medical director of addiction medicine at the Stanford University School of Medicine, wrote in an email interview. She pointed out that for those in recovery, even small amounts of alcohol could trigger cravings for more and recommended that those who are sober refrain from the drink.

Is kombucha a scam?

Given the uncertainty over kombucha's therapeutic effects, Dr. David Ludwig, professor of nutrition and pediatrics at Harvard University, said tea drinkers should pause if it's not a flavor they like. "If you're drinking this for health benefits and not enjoying the taste," Dr. Ludwig said, "I'd say rethink your drink."

But for those interested in integrating a variety of microbes into their diet, Dr. Emeran Mayer, author of "The Mind-Gut Connection," recommends doing so naturally. "I personally drink it occasionally," he said. Instead of using pills or supplements, he said, alternate different fermented foods, including sauerkraut, kimchi, cultured milk products, and, yes, kombucha.

How To Make Kombucha Tea at Home

YIELD: Makes about 1 gallon

INGREDIENTS

- 3 1/2 quarts water
- 1 cup sugar (regular granulated sugar works best)
- 8 bags black tea, green tea, or a mix (or 2 tablespoons loose tea)
- 2 cups starter tea from last batch of kombucha or store-bought kombucha (unpasteurized, neutral-flavored)
- 1 scoby per fermentation jar, homemade or purchased online
- Optional flavoring extras for bottling
- 1 to 2 cups chopped fruit
- 2 to 3 cups fruit juice

- 1 to 2 tablespoons flavored tea (like hibiscus or Earl Grey)
- 1/4 cup honey
- 2 to 4 tablespoons fresh herbs or spices

EQUIPMENTS

- Stock pot
- 1-gallon glass jar or two 2-quart glass jars
- Tightly woven cloth (like clean napkins or tea towels), covvee filters, or paper towels, to cover the jar
- Bottles: Six 16-oz glass bottles with plastic lids, swing-top bottles, or clean soda bottles
- Small funnel

INSTRUCTIONS

- Note: Avoid prolonged contact between the kombucha and metal both during and after brewing. This can affect the flavor of your kombucha and weaken the scoby over time.
- Make the tea base: Bring the water to a boil. Remove from heat and stir in the sugar to dissolve. Drop in the tea and allow it to steep until the water has cooled. Depending on the size of your pot, this will take a few hours. You can speed up the cooling process by placing the pot in an ice bath.
- Add the starter tea: Once the tea is cool, remove the tea bags or strain out the loose tea. Stir in the starter tea. (The starter tea makes the liquid acidic, which prevents

unfriendly bacteria from taking up residence in the first few days of fermentation.)

- Transfer to jars and add the scoby: Pour the mixture into a 1-gallon glass jar (or divide between two 2-quart jars, in which case you'll need 2 scobys) and gently slide the scoby into the jar with clean hands. Cover the mouth of the jar with a few layers tightly-woven cloth, coffee filters, or paper towels secured with a rubber band. (If you develop problems with gnats or fruit flies, use a tightly woven cloth or paper towels, which will do a better job keeping the insects out of your brew.)
- Ferment for 7 to 10 days: Keep the jar at room temperature, out of direct sunlight, and where it won't get jostled. Ferment for 7

to 10 days, checking the kombucha and the scoby periodically.

- It's not unusual for the scoby to float at the top, bottom, or even sideways during fermentation. A new cream-colored layer of scoby should start forming on the surface of the kombucha within a few days. It usually attaches to the old scoby, but it's ok if they separate. You may also see brown stringy bits floating beneath the scoby, sediment collecting at the bottom, and bubbles collecting around the scoby. This is all normal and signs of healthy fermentation.
- After 7 days, begin tasting the kombucha daily by pouring a little out of the jar and into a cup. When it reaches a balance of sweetness and tartness that is pleasant to you, the kombucha is ready to bottle.

- Remove the scoby: Before proceeding, prepare and cool another pot of strong tea for your next batch of kombucha, as outlined above. With clean hands, gently lift the scoby out of the kombucha and set it on a clean plate. As you do, check it over and remove the bottom layer if the scoby is getting very thick.
- Bottle the finished kombucha: Measure out your starter tea from this batch of kombucha and set it aside for the next batch. Pour the fermented kombucha (straining, if desired) into bottles using the small funnel, along with any juice, herbs, or fruit you may want to use as flavoring. Leave about a half inch of head room in each bottle. (Alternatively, infuse the kombucha with flavorings for a day or two in another covered jar, strain, and

then bottle. This makes a cleaner kombucha without "stuff" in it.)

- Carbonate and refrigerate the finished kombucha: Store the bottled kombucha at room temperature out of direct sunlight and allow 1 to 3 days for the kombucha to carbonate. Until you get a feel for how quickly your kombucha carbonates, it's helpful to keep it in plastic bottles; the kombucha is carbonated when the bottles feel rock solid. Refrigerate to stop fermentation and carbonation, and then consume your kombucha within a month.

- Make a fresh batch of kombucha: Clean the jar being used for kombucha fermentation. Combine the starter tea from your last batch of kombucha with the fresh batch of sugary tea, and pour it into the fermentation jar.

Slide the scoby on top, cover, and ferment for 7 to 10 days.

RECIPE NOTES

- Covering for the jar: Cheesecloth is not ideal because it's easy for small insects, like fruit flies, to wiggle through the layers. Use a few layers of tightly woven cloth (like clean napkins or tea towels), coffee filters, or paper towels, to cover the jar, and secure it tightly with rubber bands or twine.
- Batch Size: To increase or decrease the amount of kombucha you make, maintain the basic ratio of 1 cup of sugar, 8 bags of tea, and 2 cups starter tea per gallon batch. One scoby will ferment any size batch, though larger batches may take longer.

- Putting Kombucha on Pause: If you'll be away for 3 weeks or less, just make a fresh batch and leave it on your counter. It will likely be too vinegary to drink by the time you get back, but the scoby will be fine. For longer breaks, store the scoby in a fresh batch of the tea base with starter tea in the fridge. Change out the tea for a fresh batch every 4 to 6 weeks.
- Other Tea Options: Black tea tends to be the easiest and most reliable for the scoby to ferment into kombucha, but once your scoby is going strong, you can try branching out into other kinds. Green tea, white tea, oolong tea, or a even mix of these make especially good kombucha. Herbal teas are okay, but be sure to use at least a few bags of black tea in the mix to make sure the

scoby is getting all the nutrients it needs. Avoid any teas that contain oils, like earl grey or flavored teas.

- Avoid Prolonged Contact with Metal: Using metal utensils is generally fine, but avoid fermenting or bottling the kombucha in anything that brings them into contact with metal. Metals, especially reactive metals like aluminum, can give the kombucha a metallic flavor and weaken the scoby over time.

Troubleshooting Kombucha

It is normal for the scoby to float on the top, bottom, or sideways in the jar. It is also normal for brown strings to form below the scoby or to collect on the bottom. If your scoby develops a hole, bumps, dried patches, darker brown patches, or clear jelly-like patches, it is still fine to use. Usually these are all indicative of changes in the environment of your kitchen and not a problem with the scoby itself.

Kombucha will start off with a neutral aroma and then smell progressively more vinegary as brewing progresses. If it starts to smell cheesy, rotten, or otherwise unpleasant, this is a sign that something has gone wrong. If you see no signs of mold on the scoby, discard the liquid and begin again with fresh tea. If you do see signs of mold, discard both the scoby and the liquid and begin again with new ingredients.

A scoby will last a very long time, but it's not indestructible. If the scoby becomes black, that is a sign that it has passed its lifespan. If it develops green or black mold, it is has become infected. In both of these cases, throw away the scoby and begin again.

To prolong the life and maintain the health of your scoby, stick to the ratio of sugar, tea, starter tea, and water outlined in the recipe. You should also peel off the bottom (oldest) layer every few batches. This can be discarded, composted, used to start a new batch of kombucha, or given to a friend to start their own.

If you're ever in doubt about whether there is a problem with your scoby, just continue brewing batches but discard the kombucha they make. If there's a problem, it will get worse over time and become very apparent. If it's just a natural aspect of the scoby, then it will stay consistent from batch to batch and the kombucha is fine for drinking

Conclusion

Kombucha drink is consumed worldwide as a homemade refreshing beverage and it is also commercially sold by some companies. Different tea leaf varieties, amounts of sugar, fermentation time, and composition of tea fungus may account for differences in composition and therefore also the biological activities of kombucha tea. There is still a dispute over the beneficial effects of kombucha drink. There has been no evidence published to date on the biological activities of kombucha in human trials. All the biological activities have been investigated using animal experimental models. Toxicity reports on kombucha drink are very rare and scattered. Toxicity must be evaluated thoroughly using modern procedures. Tea fungus is an excellent example of biofilm and studies on its cellulose chemistry must be encouraged. Cellulose in tea fungus can be used as a successful alternative to traditional cellulose in various applications. Although kombucha tea cannot be granted official health claims at this time, it can be recognized as an important part of a sound diet. Not exactly a traditional beverage, kombucha tea is now regarded as a "health" drink, a source of pharmacologically active molecules, an important member of the antioxidant food group, and a functional food with potential beneficial health properties. Research on kombucha demonstrating its beneficial effects and their mechanisms will most likely continue to increase substantially in the next few years. It is apparent that kombucha tea is a source of a wide range of bioactive components that are digested, absorbed, and metabolized by the body, and exert their effects at the cellular level. Kombucha tea's current status as a functional food as summarized in this review, lends credibility to what has been believed by kombucha tea drinkers for a long time.

Printed in Great Britain
by Amazon